I0424716

Wellness Group Toolkit

Ideas and Exercises for Support and/or Wellness Groups

Carmen Freeman, MS, CHT

Copyright © 2010 Carmen Freeman, MS, CHT
All rights reserved.

ISBN: 1453679901
ISBN-13: 9781453679906
Library of Congress Control Number: 2010910003

Dedication

This book is dedicated to:

The Boulder MS Wellness Group, especially Lynne Barnett, Shireen Miller, and Anna Scott.

The kindred souls who attended various workshops I facilitated, and who trusted me to challenge them to embrace wellness—despite the "evidence of the senses."

David Luce, MD, my doctor-brother-friend—a physician who truly practices patient-centered medicine, and who provides the data and tools for us to heal ourselves.

Ed Freeman, PhD, my husband of almost four decades—and the love of my life. You are a wonderful blend of intellect and spirituality, a "quiet giant," who *sees* me and supports me in all endeavors.

My daughters, Isis and China, fierce young women possessing many gifts and endless compassion.

My mother, who first modeled the ability to be self-defined, despite the circumstances.

Sri Gary, who consistently, lovingly points me in the direction of the Friend.

Physically challenged people, who seek to live creative, balanced, authentic, and empowered lives—no matter what!

Table of Contents

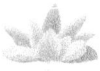

The *I* in illness is isolation, and the crucial letters in wellness are *we*.

—*author unknown*—

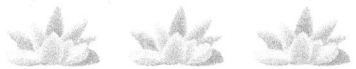

Preface

Everyone who is born holds dual citizenship, in the kingdom of the well and in the kingdom of the sick. Although we all prefer to use only the good passport, sooner or later each of us is obliged, at least for a spell, to identify ourselves as citizens of that other place.

—Susan Sontag, *Illness as Metaphor*, 1977

In the late seventies, shortly after the birth of my second daughter, I received a diagnosis of "probable multiple sclerosis." I had been hospitalized due to a bout with optic neuritis, in addition to other symptoms that had surfaced: dropped right foot, balance, and proprioception issues, pain, numbness, extreme fatigue, and a sensation of shock that traveled down my right arm. I had completed an excruciating battery of tests, finally submitting to a spinal tap, the results of which confirmed the tentative diagnosis.

I left the hospital, not with the usual prescription for prednisone (common for that time) and a grim outlook, but with a resolve to study the disease, and more importantly, to engage a course of self-study as I navigated the landscape of the physically challenged. I had received a great undergraduate education from UCLA and had established a daily discipline of meditation several years prior, so I felt well equipped for the journey into the unknown that seemed to be unfolding.

The road warped, twisted, and turned in many directions as I sought answers to daily dilemmas that arose pertaining to my care, as well as the care, feeding, and nurturing of the two beautiful daughters with whom I was entrusted.

Shortly after my husband, Ed, finished his PhD, I returned to graduate school, earning an ed-psych degree, with a specialization in educational computing, where I learned about curriculum development and, through classes in both education and psychology, developed skills as a trainer. Shortly after completing this, we moved to Boulder, Colorado, where Ed played a role in developing new technologies. Boulder also happened to be one of the first cities to receive the Magnetic Resonance Imaging (MRI) machines, and I was one of the first patients to experience brain scans via this new equipment.

It was here that I received a definite diagnosis of MS. After my second diagnosis, I decided to attend my first MS support group meeting—which changed everything.

The meeting was filled with people who lived their lives from the perspective of "suffering with MS," as if this defined their existence. Sugary, unhealthy refreshments were served, and some of the participants smoked cigarettes. Many of the members exhibited defeatist attitudes, voicing numerous complaints. I had compassion and didn't set out to judge the other people in the room, but for me, the atmosphere was downright depressing. Within two days, I had an exacerbation, which I attributed to the infectious depression looming in that meeting. I vowed never to go back. If I was going to connect with other people with MS, I needed to seek those who were interested in mapping their illness into a larger view about their life. I silently made a promise to help build a community of like-minded people.

A few years later, I began training as a transpersonal hypnotherapist, specializing in physical challenges. After thousands of hours of training, I became certified and began my career. In the early nineties, I owned a growing practice and began teaching workshops entitled "Physically Challenged and Empowered" for people with MS. These workshops grew into the Multiple Sclerosis and Empowered support group, which grew into the MS Wellness Group that met once a month in Boulder, Colorado, for thirteen years. In addition to facilitating this group, I was a guest facilitator for other "support" groups, taught various workshops, and helped create "wellness conferences" for the MS Society. I created a national women's retreat and facilitated workshops for other organizations. I was honored with several recognitions for this work, including an MS Achievement Award.

Over the course of many years, I acquired or developed various tools for facilitating groups of individuals that shared a desire to see themselves as more than their illnesses. These courageous individuals saw me as "one of them," someone who understands that we are not a disease—but rather, we are whole people, who are challenged by our bodies, in a world where everyone is challenged by something. I was given permission to occasionally guide these individuals to places not usually ventured within the confines of traditional support groups, and was acknowledged by the willing, cooperative community we created during the ensuing years. For this, I am grateful.

It is my greatest wish that the contents of these pages serve all who venture here—all who seek to embrace the wellness paradigm.

Introduction

The last of one's freedoms is to choose one's attitude in any given circumstance.

—Victor Frankl

I reconnected with a friend when she was in the fourth stage of cancer. We had a lengthy conversation, during which I learned that the only grain her body could tolerate was quinoa[1]; and while most people have never eaten quinoa, I was very familiar with it and considered myself to be the "quinoa queen." As we continued our conversation, I discovered that she had many dietary needs and restrictions, and she wanted wholesome, organic food. Prior to and during my thirty years with MS, I had studied many dietary programs and lived with various healthy diet regimes. Since I already had an understanding about healing foods, it seemed natural to become a member of the "food detail." I began cooking for her on Mondays and Thursdays, taking her the finished creations in the afternoon or evening.

While it took quite a bit of work to shop for the foods, prep them, cook, package everything, and drive thirty minutes or more to deliver her meals, I began to look forward to these visits. Upon arrival, someone from hospice usually opened the door. Their presence, plus the diagnosis of "fourth stage cancer," indicated the limitation in prognosis for my friend. The meaning was clear: she would not recover. Yet, despite all this, she was boldly asserting her right to embrace the concept of wellness. This was evident everywhere within her home from the healing affirmations posted in conspicuous places to the alternative substances she was ingesting, her request for organic and healing foods, and the attention to detail in creating a holistic healing atmosphere, etc.

Clearly, some might have labeled her behaviors as indicative of the state of denial, and under different circumstances, I might have been inclined to agree. However, my

---

1 Quinoa: a "grain-like" complete protein originating in South America. Usually eaten as a grain, it is actually a seed of a plant similar to beets and chard. It is easy to digest, is gluten-free, and contains all the amino acids.

friend repeatedly demonstrated that she understood the prognosis but chose to embrace wellness as a lifestyle—to the very end of her life.

I decided to participate in this vision. It was a blessing to be with her, and it validated a personal message that I had embodied for over thirty years: wellness is not necessarily the absence of symptoms; rather, it is a state of consciousness and set of practices wherein one strives for wholeness and balance, despite the diagnosis or symptoms. This became the matrix for the foundation of the Boulder MS Wellness Group.

A wellness group empowers and supports those who wish to live a more balanced life—body, mind and spirit—even if physical challenges are present. This book provides questions, thoughts, and exercises that will assist you in facilitating this type of group or introducing elements of wellness practices into more traditional support groups. You can use as much, or as little, of these pages, as you like. It's called a "toolkit" because you can simply remove and use whatever is needed to get the job done.

If you are looking for a guidebook for starting a support group, keep looking. That is not what I've attempted to do here. There are plenty of books that address methods for creating self-help groups, and numerous societies that train potential facilitators to coordinate affiliated groups. These can be researched via the Internet.

When I began the Boulder MS Wellness Group, I was never interested in merely "supporting"; I was interested in empowering people to embrace the concept of wellness "despite the evidence of the senses," and the disempowering messages that bombarded them once they had a diagnosis of disease. I wanted to "infect" others with my viewpoint, which was that "I have MS, but MS doesn't have me!" Despite the challenges of disease, I always knew that the disease did not define me unless I consented to that viewpoint…and I did not consent.

If you've been diagnosed with an illness and are facilitating a support group, or are charged with facilitating a group of physically challenged individuals and want to move beyond old paradigms regarding coping skills, drug therapy, and traditional support groups, the "toolkit" has something to offer. If you want to climb out of the box and experiment with viewpoints that may empower you and members of your group, here you will find food and water for your care and feeding.

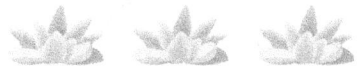

How to Use This Book

As time goes by, you will come to realize that groups are living organisms. They have an ebb and flow, they breathe in and out, they eat, they discard, they give birth, and when their lifespan is complete, they expire. Within the lifetime of the group, there will be times when people show up just to talk, making other types of activities inappropriate. There will be times when the group seems to take on a life of its own—when the creativity of its members is in full swing, or conversely, when inspiration is stifled. There will be times when members show up with immediate survival needs or a crisis of some type or the exhaustion of living day-to-day. There are also times when everyone shows up ready to charge ahead.

Be open to the needs of the group in the moment, because if the issues that emerge are not acknowledged, members may become disempowered, rather than empowered.

During the lifespan of your group, many needs will arise. These needs may be divided into three categories. First, there will be a need for members to simply "show up" and tell their current story. The facilitator should pay attention as members convene for the meeting, noticing the subject matter of side conversations, as members greet each other upon entrance to the room. If a particular theme seems to dominate (i.e. worsening condition, diagnosis information, some form of loss or grievance), it may be a signal that the evening's activities should revolve around more traditional support group activities—talking and listening in a safe environment. Likewise, there may be cause for celebration (remission, successful treatment, new support, etc.), in which case sharing during the entire meeting is also appropriate. It may be the case that group members prefer this format most of the time, reserving special activities for times when a change is temporarily needed.

Another need that will become evident for wellness groups is the need to define, redefine, and/or support the idea of "wellness." This is where wellness groups diverge from more traditional support groups. Most support groups do not place an emphasis on wellness, preferring instead to simply offer nonjudgmental support for its members. This is a formula that has worked very well for a long time. However, an emphasis on wellness can create a place where members who are usually very aware of their illness can focus more on living a life of wholeness, embracing and acknowledging themselves as whole beings, despite physical symptoms and challenges.

It can be a powerful experience to "show up" and embrace wellness, despite one's diagnosis; and to do this in a room full of like-minded individuals reinforces this viewpoint, creating another powerful experience—that of beginning to internalize the idea that wellness can exist in a diseased body, and can be accessed through daily life. I've been privileged to witness this transformative realization many times—at conferences, the support group I facilitated, and with the support groups where I was a guest facilitator. In order for members to access this idea of wellness despite outward appearances, they have to embrace a larger viewpoint about who they are—and that viewpoint elevates them to the realm of body, mind, and spirit.

The activities in this book are designed to subtly support this viewpoint, as well as a "third need"—the need to maintain the group as fresh, innovative, and supportive of the growth of members, as they engage their personal journey with challenging circumstances.

Group Format

The Boulder MS Wellness Group format usually followed variations of the following protocol:

> ### FORMAT A
>
> - Check-in via a choice of questions
> - Group meditation or contemplative technique
> - A chosen wellness-enhancing activity
> - Several minutes of sharing about the wellness activity
> - Close

FORMAT B

- Group meditation or contemplative technique
- Members share briefly about their current life experience, followed by answering a chosen question (creates an open sharing opportunity, and an opportunity for members to map their current experience into a larger viewpoint)
- A chosen wellness-enhancing activity
- Several minutes of sharing about the wellness activity
- Close

FORMAT C

- Group meditation or contemplative technique
- Open-ended check-in and discussion/sharing
- Close

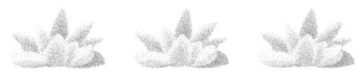

Beginnings

A Word about Safety and Trust

There are several ways to establish safety and trust in a group setting. For the purposes of the wellness group, we will focus on two of them: Group Guidelines and Telling Your Story.

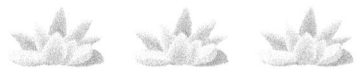

Group Guidelines

There are as many different group guidelines as there are groups! Several examples exist via the Internet, or if you are facilitating a group for one of the research societies, guidelines may be provided to you. If you are free to do so, you may also create your own guidelines or ask the group to create their personalized set of guidelines.

Although different, guidelines usually contain some of the following elements:

Confidentiality: whatever happens in the group stays in the group.

Speaking: one person speaks at a time.

Sharing: everyone is encouraged to tell their story, but this is optional.

Advice: don't give advice unless asked, but do share experiences.

Acceptance: everyone is accepted for who they are.

Discussion: no cross-talk or discussing anyone not present.

Stay in the Present: share about your current experience; don't stay in the past.

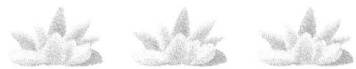

Telling Your Story

Whether I'm facilitating my own group, guest facilitating for another group, offering a workshop at a conference, or working with a ballroom full of people, I often begin by telling my story. Because I am physically challenged, it allows participants to understand that I am one of them—that I am not an expert who will be "talking at" them, but rather, I live a life where physical challenge and wellness comingle.

When the facilitator shares his or her story, it also gives permission for participants to share. As we acknowledge our vulnerabilities and strengths, others are more willing to acknowledge their own. The simple act of telling your story breaks the ice and allows for trust to build in a natural way.

Sometimes, before we begin with the personal stories, I request the group to sit quietly with eyes closed, and together as a group we hold the intention of creating a safe space for whatever needs to happen at the meeting.

As you continue to meet and the group members become more acquainted, the safety and trust quotient should naturally increase.

Contemplative Practices

*The ultimate value of life depends upon awareness and the
power of contemplation rather than upon mere survival.*

—Aristotle

*All that Is, like You
Breathes in, breathes out.
The more it releases
The more it takes in.
Much talk about healing
Will stifle you.
Be still and breathe.*

—Haven Trevino, *The Tao of Healing*

The Role of Contemplative Practice

It is beneficial to engage some type of contemplative practice, within the first
few minutes of any group gathering—either before or directly after a group check-in.
Checking in can be defined as the process of creating space for each person to speak
his or her current experience. It can begin with a question (see Openings—20 Empowering Questions), or can take the form of simple, casual statements about what's
going on in the individual's life.

Using contemplative practices before the checking-in process can create a more
focused viewpoint regarding what each person expresses. I've found that members
tend to be more mindful about what they are sharing when we begin this way, whereas

members are more emotional about whatever is present in their lives when contemplative practice is second on the agenda.

There is a place for both approaches—both states of consciousness—and it is the job of the facilitator to be sensitive about which approach is needed at any given time, based upon your attunement to the group. Regarding when to use each approach, perhaps an example will suffice.

Let's say that on this particular night, members arrive and spontaneously begin sharing as they enter the room. One member looks particularly distraught and begins sharing about his or her exacerbation, flare-up, or alarming symptoms. Other members are listening; some are even expressing empathy or similar experiences. Now might not be the time to cut this sharing short, forcing a contemplative exercise, when the natural order seems to be to go with the flow—allowing full expression of the experience. Instead, relax, take a deep breath, and listen for the ebb in the conversation, which may signal an opportunity to introduce the contemplative practice. Scheduling contemplative practices *this way* may create an opening to view exacerbated symptoms from a different perspective.

On the other hand, if group members enter the room without such an urgent, obvious need, the facilitator can choose to immediately begin with a contemplative practice, followed by a period of checking in.

In essence, facilitating a wellness group is much like conducting an orchestra—working with the personalities and instruments in the room, along with the structure provided by the sheet music. The facilitator is sensitive to the needs and personalities present, within the container of flexible structure.

Below is a non-exhaustive smorgasbord of contemplative practices from which to choose. Try different ones, and notice the effect on the group—always paying attention to group feedback. You may find that some practices do not work for your group. On the other hand, you may find that certain ones work well at distinct times, while others work better at other times. Or, you may stay with one or two practices. The choice is up to you and the individuals with whom you are meeting.

Over time, you may notice that contemplative practices have some of the following effects:

- Increased sense of well-being
- Decreased stress levels
- Increased ability to observe stressors and their effects on the body
- Increased ability to choose how to respond to events, emotions, stressors, and relationships
- Decreased judgmental-ism and other energy-draining emotions, accompanied by an increase in compassion for self and others

• More self-understanding, accompanied by greater focus—which can enhance decision making
• A growing understanding that one's life is greater than one's physical symptoms

My daily spiritual practice revolves around Surat Shabda Yoga, or the Light and Sound Teachings. However, during the past thirty-eight years, I've experienced several forms of contemplative practice, and I believe that for every type of person, or personality, there is a contemplative practice that will be appealing. Therefore, I have offered a variety of techniques to the group, allowing members who do not have a personal practice to find what was comfortable for them.

It is also a good idea to listen to feedback and adjust contemplative exercises as needed, or provide variety based upon the mood of the group. Over time, by paying conscious attention, this becomes second nature. As a group facilitator, it is advantageous to develop a practice of one's own and to encourage group members to create a daily discipline of their own choosing, which can be practiced at home.

Listed below are simple practices that can be used by your group:

Mindfulness Meditation

Begin by creating an environment that is free from unnecessary noise and distractions. Instruct each member to sit comfortably, with feet on the floor, with the body in a relaxed, upright position. Group members who are mobile via motorized chair or requiring different positions to facilitate unobstructed breathing and/or swallowing should choose a position that allows freedom from distress, yet enables them to participate in the group practice.

Begin by closing the eyes and focusing on the breath. As you do so, you may notice some tension in the body. It's OK to notice this tension. In fact, you may label it, saying to yourself, "Oh, I'm experiencing some tension in my body." Then, try to simply relax, release the tension, and return to an awareness of the breath.

Just settle in now, and notice that the body "breathes itself."

Whatever sounds you hear or sensations you experience can simply be noticed for what they are, and labeled ("I'm hearing the sound of -blank-"), followed by a gentle return to an awareness of the breath.

After the amount of time agreed upon by the group or requested by the facilitator (starting with five or ten minutes, possibly increasing to fifteen or twenty minutes over time), the facilitator requests members to gradually return their awareness to the room. Allow three to five minutes for this transition.

In the beginning, it might also be a good idea to allow time to talk about the group practice. Members might want to express that it was easy or hard; or questions might arise as to whether they were engaging the practice correctly. Whatever questions arise, remind fellow practitioners to simply allow for an awareness of the experiences that draw the attention, label or acknowledge them, and gently return to awareness of the breath.

Eyes Open

A variation of mindfulness meditation can be practiced with eyes open. Instruct members to softly gaze or gently focus on a point several inches in front of their nose, or a point on the floor. All other instructions are the same.

If the eyes water or members are distracted by something visually, the instructions are to simply acknowledge or label the experience, then gently return to a soft gaze or focus, followed by a return to the breath.

Bells, Gongs & Crystal Bowls

During the years of facilitating meetings, meditations and workshops, bells, gongs, or crystal bowls were frequently used to begin and/or end the meditation. Bells and small gongs or cymbals can be purchased in stores that sell meditation supplies or Asian arts, and certain bookstores. Sometimes members have reported an appreciation for the sounds produced by these instruments as a wordless signal to begin or end. Sometimes, there is also an appreciation of a sound that one can "follow" into meditation or contemplation.

The clear and penetrating sound emanating from a crystal bowl can help facilitate a relaxation response. I often use them as instruments for initiating a group contemplative practice. The bowl is not struck like a percussion instrument, but rather a cushioned mallet is pulled around the circumference of the opening of the bowl, which creates a lasting harmonic reverberation capable of penetrating deep into the body and mind. Members respond to this reverberation by easily and naturally following this sound into the contemplative exercise that has been chosen.

Music

Group members may sometimes want to simply sit with eyes closed while listening to relaxing music. While this cannot necessarily be categorized as a contemplative practice, it can be relaxing and stress- relieving for members, and doesn't seem to disturb those group members who have an established practice.

Look for music in the "ambient" category, or choose relaxing classical or spiritual music. Some beginning suggestions for group music are listed in the resources section of this book.

Contemplation

Contemplation is often defined as "thoughtful observation." While some forms of meditation aim to still the mind as a goal, contemplation gives the mind something to do. During the practice of contemplation, you choose a subject almost as if you are choosing a destination. For example, if you were to contemplate Los Angeles, you might start with the destination itself, exploring Los Angeles from various heights, locations, and time periods, as well as the demographics of Los Angeles. You might explore via roads or flight; or, arrival to versus departure from the city. You might examine the neighborhoods from the suburbs to the inner city. Using the practice of contemplation, you might follow all the pathways of thought regarding everything about Los Angeles.

Likewise, during a contemplation practice, pick the subject matter and explore all angles and pathways regarding that subject. The benefit of this type of practice is that you arrive at an understanding of the ins and outs, ups and downs, and all characteristics of the subject, because you have thoroughly examined from all angles via "thoughtful observation." Contemplation is a useful practice for people who are physically challenged in that it may: a) lessen the fear and/or anxiety around the subject matter that is contemplated, b) uncover realizations, information, and emotions which can be further examined, c) decrease stress levels and contribute to more self-awareness.

In a group setting, I have used two types of contemplation exercises: 1) subjects that arise spontaneously during the process of checking in, and 2) subjects that arise during the course of the meeting.

Subjects that arise during check-in

Check-ins provide opportunities for members to share the inner workings of their lives. Sometimes we allow our check-in periods to be free-form, in that we simply sit listening while members share whatever is on their minds. Often, the subject to be contemplated emerges naturally by listening to common themes that arise during our time of checking in.

It is the facilitator's job to simply be aware of any emerging issues that beg contemplation. Over time, you may become more able to ascertain when to put aside any planned agenda, and follow rather than lead the group into an exploration of the subjects that have arisen.

Let's use an actual example of a subject that arose for the Boulder group. Years ago during a meeting, a woman who was mobile via wheelchair and who had been service-oriented prior to her diagnosis, raised this question: "How can I serve others, now that I'm no longer ambulatory?" The subject was service; we all contemplated what "service" meant for us at that point in our lives, examining the concept of service from all angles. After ten or fifteen minutes, we returned our awareness to the room and had a revealing discussion about service. Some people expressed ways they could physically participate in service organizations, while others accessed more spiritual ways of providing service: prayer; private, silent blessings; and open, attentive presence and listening with someone who needed to be heard.

Despite the perception that this contemplation required some work, an air of peacefulness prevailed afterwards. All participants were satisfied that, if the need to be of service surfaced, even though our bodies were differently-abled, many options were available.

A variation is to listen during an open-ended check-in. After everyone has had their turn, ask members to contemplate something they noticed about themselves, or their experience, during their time of sharing. Closing their eyes and remembering what they shared can help facilitate honing in on the subject matter that would be suitable for each person.

<u>Subjects that arise during the course of the meeting</u>

Sometimes, the subject for contemplation shows up naturally and spontaneously as an experience or thought pattern that is shared by members of the group. While this may occur during the group check-in, it can also occur as the meeting proceeds, as members engage in other activities. For example, individuals might complain about being "unseen" or misunderstood. If you observe that several people seem affected by this thought, or are in agreement about this experience, designating this (the idea of feeling "unseen") as a subject of contemplation, could be undertaken in the following way:

1) First, create a sense of safety by asking the group to hold the intention of creating a safe space for the contemplation, or use another method of your choosing to create safety.

2) Ask members to contemplate the concept of being unseen, examining it from all angles. If a particular thought or emotion regarding the subject arises, instruct them to follow that thought and notice where it takes them (i.e. subsequent thoughts, resolution, or greater realizations). You might also ask participants to seek the *source* of any emotional response to that thought or construct. Allow ten minutes or so for the exercise.

3) Follow up with a period of sharing the experience, for those who would like to share. Always offer the option to speak about the experience—or to remain silent.

Relaxation Training (including Progressive Relaxation)

Relaxation training (or relaxation technique) is defined as: *any method, process, procedure, or activity that helps a person to relax; to attain a state of increased calmness; or otherwise reduce levels of anxiety, stress or anger.* Relaxation techniques are often employed as one element of a wider stress management program and can decrease muscle tension, lower the blood pressure, and slow heart and breath rates, among other health benefits (Wikipedia).

Progressive relaxation is a technique for reducing anxiety by alternately tensing and relaxing the muscles. This method was developed by physician Edmund Jacobson in the early 1920s, when it was argued that since muscular tension accompanies anxiety, you can reduce anxiety by learning how to relax muscular tension.

During progressive relaxation, muscles are tensed and then relaxed in a progressive ascending or descending order (starting with the head, neck, face, shoulders, arms, back of the arms, chest, abdomen, legs, and feet, etc.), or in the opposite order, starting with the feet. With eyes closed, a tension or squeezing is purposefully created by the participant in a given muscle group for approximately several seconds, and then released and relaxed for several seconds, before proceeding to the next muscle group. The facilitator may use soft background music or choose to only use soft, gentle voice commands.

Since most illnesses and physical challenges are exacerbated by stress, including these techniques periodically can provide immediate benefits, as well as stress management training for group members.

Here is a general script for facilitating one type of relaxation for the group.

Progressive Muscle Relaxation

[NOTE: If you are dealing with a group that is differently-abled, mention the following: "If you are unable to control certain muscle groups, simply 'think tension,' when you hear the suggestion to tense the muscles. Likewise, simply 'think release' when you hear the suggestion to release; and follow along with all other muscle groups."

Make yourself comfortable in your chair, or lying on the floor.

Close your eyes, and begin by taking in three (3) deep, cleansing breaths…

Now breathe normally…and allow yourself to relax a bit more…with each breath…

Bring your attention to your toes and feet…Feel your arches, the tops and soles of your feet…your heels…and all areas of your feet…

Now, tense your feet and toes…curl them, or make them tense…notice how it feels to hold tension in your toes and feet…
Hold that tension…hold…hold… [Hold to a count of four (4).]
Now inhale…and as you exhale, release all the tension …
Notice what it feels like to release the tension in your toes and feet.

Bring your attention to your calves and lower legs...feel your calves, the backs and fronts of your lower legs...

Now, tense your calves and lower legs...Notice how it feels to hold tension in this area...
Hold that tension...hold...hold... [Hold to a count of four (4).]
Now inhale...and as you exhale, release all the tension...
Notice what it feels like to release all the tension in your calves and lower legs...

Bring your attention to your thighs and buttocks...feel the backs and fronts of your thighs, along with your buttocks...

Now, tense this whole area...Notice how it feels to hold tension here...
Hold that tension...hold...hold... [Hold to a count of four (4).]
Now inhale...and as you exhale, release all the tension...from your buttocks...from your thighs...
Notice what it feels like to release all the tension in this area...

Bring your attention to your abdomen and lower back...Feel your abdomen, and become aware of your lower back...

Now, tense your abdomen and lower back...Squeeze them together, pulling your navel toward your spine...Notice how it feels to hold the tension in this area...
Hold that tension...hold...hold... [Hold to a count of four (4).]
Now inhale...and as you exhale, release all the tension from your abdomen and lower back...
Notice how it feels to release all this tension...to just let it go...
Notice how it feels for the abdomen and lower back to be totally relaxed...

Now, bring your attention to your right arm and hand...Notice any tension that is currently there...

Now, tense your right arm and make a fist with your hand... Squeeze your fist tighter, and contract or tense your right arm...Notice how it feels to hold the tension in this area...
Now, hold that tension...hold...hold...Squeeze tighter... [Hold to a count of four (4).]
Now inhale...and as you exhale, release all the tension from your right arm and hand...
Release your fist...release your entire right arm...let them go limp at your side...
Notice how it feels to release all this tension...
Notice how it feels for the right arm and hand to be totally relaxed...

Now, bring your attention to your left arm and hand...Notice any tension that is currently there...

Now, tense your left arm and make a fist with your hand...Squeeze your fist tighter, and contract or tense your left arm...Notice how it feels to hold the tension in this area...
Hold that tension...hold...hold...Squeeze tighter... [Hold to a count of four (4).]
Now inhale...and as you exhale, release all the tension from your left arm and hand...
Release your fist...release your entire left arm...let them go limp at your side...
Notice how it feels to release all this tension...
Notice how it feels for the left arm and hand to be totally relaxed...

Bring your attention to your upper back and shoulder blades...Notice any tension that is currently there...

Now, tense your upper back and shoulder blades...Squeeze your shoulder blades, squeeze your upper back...Notice how it feels to hold the tension here...
Hold that tension...hold...hold...Squeeze tighter... [Hold to a count of four (4).]
Now inhale...and as you exhale, release all the tension from your upper back and shoulder blades...Just release, relax, and let go of any tension...
Notice how it feels to release all this tension...
Notice how it feels for the upper back and shoulder blades to be totally relaxed...

Bring your attention to your shoulders...

Now, squeeze your shoulders...Squeeze them up toward your neck and head in a tense shrug...Shrug your shoulders even more...Notice how it feels to hold the tension in this area...
Hold that tension...hold...hold...Squeeze tighter... [Hold to a count of four (4).]
Now inhale...and as you exhale, release all the tension from shoulders...
Notice how it feels to release all this tension...
Notice how it feels for the shoulders to be totally relaxed...

Now, bring your attention to your neck, chin, and jaws...Notice any tension that is currently there...

Now, tense your neck, chin, and jaws...Squeeze them all together...Notice how it feels to hold the tension in this area...
Hold that tension...hold...hold...Squeeze tighter... [Hold to a count of four (4).]

Now inhale…and as you exhale, release all the tension from your neck, chin, and jaws…
Notice how it feels to release all this tension…
Notice how it feels for the neck, chin, and jaws to be totally relaxed…

Now, bring your attention to your face…Notice any tension you are already holding there…

Now, squeeze and tense your face…
Hold that tension…hold…hold…Squeeze tighter… [Hold to a count of four (4)]
Now inhale…and as you exhale, release all the tension from your face…just let it go… and totally relax your facial muscles…
Notice how it feels to release all this tension…
Notice how it feels for the face to be totally relaxed…

Take a moment or two to sit (lie) here, just breathing…in a totally relaxed body…and when you are ready, open your eyes…

Group Visualization

Here is a variation of a relaxing group visualization I have often used with wellness groups and conference participants, which has elements of progressive relaxation, yet engages more of the senses (visual and kinesthetic, rather than kinesthetic alone). It works well with relaxing, ambient music but is equally effective without music. It should be read with a slow, hypnotic, relaxed pace.

Golden, Healing Light Visualization

Begin by closing your eyes, and taking in three deep, cleansing breaths. Relax into your chair (the floor). On the next exhale, give yourself a command to relax even more deeply...

Now imagine a glowing ball of healing, light energy...at the base of your feet...And this ball of energy also radiates a very gentle, comforting warmth...

As you watch, some of the healing light energy enters your feet...caressing your toes...relaxing them...And this energy enters the rest of your feet...your arches... your heels...the tops of your feet...all the way to your ankles...so that now, your feet are entirely engulfed by the warmth and energy of this healing light...and they are completely relaxed, yet energized...both...at the same time...

Next, this energy enters your lower legs...calves...fronts and backs of the lower legs...and you easily and naturally watch and feel as all tension simply melts away... You feel the warmth...you see the light...that is engulfing your legs and feet...and they are totally relaxed...yet, they are also energized...

As you continue to watch and feel this energy that's gracing your body with healing and warmth, the light enters, relaxes and heals your knees...your thighs...upper and lower...and it moves into your hips and buttocks...which are now enveloped by light and warmth...healing light and warmth...

Then, this healing light energy moves upward...into your abdomen and lower back... and as you watch and breathe... your abdomen simply relaxes and releases...And as you continue to simply breathe, this relaxation and healing deepens...and on the next exhale, you can easily relax even more deeply...knowing that this healing light is guided by an innate intelligence. It knows exactly what to do...

Next, this light energy moves upward still...into your upper back and chest area... relaxing and releasing all tension there...as you watch and feel it melt away...

The light then moves into your shoulder blades…and the tissue around your shoulder blades…and notice how it feels when these areas are completely relaxed…yet alive with energy…

Then, as you watch, this healing energy moves into your neck…front and back…and into your throat…as all tension melts into the golden light…

And then, something interesting happens…

This golden, healing light energy splits in two and moves into your shoulders…and down both arms…relaxing and releasing them…as it flows into your hands… And, as you continue to watch and feel the light, it moves into your hands…visibly filling and relaxing your fingers and all the tissues in your hands…

Continue watching…as it flows out the tips of your fingers…See the light flowing out the tips of your fingers…feel the sensation of that…

Now, as you gaze at your body…and feel the relaxing sensations of your body…you are completely filled and surrounded by golden light…from the neck down…

Now bring your attention back to the place where the light split…the area of your neck…From here, the healing light travels up and into your head area…surrounding and engulfing your chin…your jaw and cheeks…your mouth…the area around your nose…See your entire eye area bathing in this golden energy…

See your forehead relax and release all tension…watch the light envelope the back and top of your head…

Then, watch and feel this healing light energy caressing and healing the scalp…and each individual hair follicle or pore…every inch of scalp…and then notice the energy begin to pour out of the top of your head…

And oh, what a wonderful sensation… [Pause for a count of four (4).]

Just pause and breathe it in…

And as you simply continue to relax and breathe, notice that your whole body is now completely surrounded, protected, and filled with this golden, healing light energy.

Breathe it in and bask in it for a moment or two…feeling totally relaxed, yet energized…at the same time.

Know that you can return to this feeling anytime you visualize this golden, healing energy…continue to breathe and bask in it's warmth…and when you are ready, slowly open your eyes.

I have found that the greatest help in meeting any problem is to know where you yourself stand. That is, to have in words what you believe and are acting from.

—William Faulkner

Openings—20 Empowering Questions

[Note: While the questions listed below do not necessarily address specific problems, they open a dialogue for members to explore their feelings and beliefs about various subjects that may impact individual wellness ideas and practices. Refer to the section **"How to Use This Book"** for suggestions about using the questions with your group.]

1. Today, in this moment, what is the most valuable lesson your illness or challenge is teaching or has taught you?
2. Close your eyes for a moment and imagine you have a "wellness bag." Into this bag you've placed physical objects, attitudes, and practices that help you increase your "wellness factor" at any time. Now, pull something out of this bag, share it with us, and tell us how it serves you.
3. If your illness is a teacher, what is it teaching you?
4. What is the biggest day-to-day challenge you face, and who are the allies you can call upon to assist and empower you?
5. Here is a quote by a man named Joseph Ortega y Gasset: "Tell me to what you pay attention, and I will tell you who you are." Tell us to what you pay attention, and how it serves you.
6. Complete these sentences: "I feel the most vulnerable when… I feel the most empowered when…" What have you noticed about yourself simply by answering these questions?
7. What I really want people to know about me—as I journey through this [illness, challenge] is…

8. Imagine you are travelling on a winding road and you come to a crossroad, where you meet an older version of yourself. What does your older and wiser self say to you?

9. Complete these thoughts: "I know I'm broken because... (and) I know I'm beautiful [or choose attractive or whole] because..."

10. How do you feel about the following statement: Pain is an experience everyone encounters, but suffering is a state of consciousness.

11. Each of us knows there is something in our life that detracts from our wellness. These can be habits, thoughts, people, etc.; or a *lack* of health-enhancing habits, thoughts, or people. It can be powerful to articulate these areas of our lives that need balancing, and coupled with an articulation of the remedy, a healthier lifestyle can be jump-started. Take a moment to assess the areas of your life that need adjustment, and share one of these with us, as well as the solution.

12. Tell us about a recent incident you experienced that seemed to be negative or restricting, at first glance, but which turned out to be a blessing in disguise.

13. When you're having a rough day, what do you do to create a shift in your experience? When this doesn't seem to be enough, what do you do next?

14. What follows is a quote by Caroline Myss, a famous medical intuitive. I'm going to read the quote, as food for thought, and then I'd like us to assess how we feel about it, and respond: "We are very presumptuous to negate the possibility that an illness may be a gift. It's a neutral experience, is what I'm trying to say. It should be viewed in some regard as no different than any other experience." What do you think?

15. There is a quote by Louise Hays, which goes like this: "Every thought we think is creating our future." If this is true, what future have you been creating with your thoughts, and how do these thoughts affect your wellness?

16. On a scale of 1 to 10, how are you feeling [choose "physically" or "emotionally"] today, and why? What needs to happen next?

17. Victor Frankl, who survived the concentration camps during the Holocaust, is known to have said: "The last of the human freedoms is to choose one's attitude in any given set of circumstances." Tell us about a recent circumstance for which you are aware that you choose the wrong attitude. How does this realization serve you now?

18. Helen Keller said: "It is a terrible thing to see and have no vision." In the present moment, what is the vision for your life?

19. What is the gift others see when they witness the way you live with your challenge?

20. Anais Nin said: "We don't see things as they are, we see them as we are." What would you say is characteristic about how you see your illness/challenge, and what does that say about your nature, in this moment?

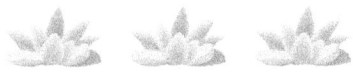

Group Exercises

On the following pages, you'll find samples of exercises that have been used in support groups, wellness groups, conference workshops, and workshops for such organizations as senior centers and advocacy groups. In some cases, there are worksheets, for which permission is granted to create copies. All copyrights remain the property of the author, but feel free to use the worksheets with your group.

Personal Values

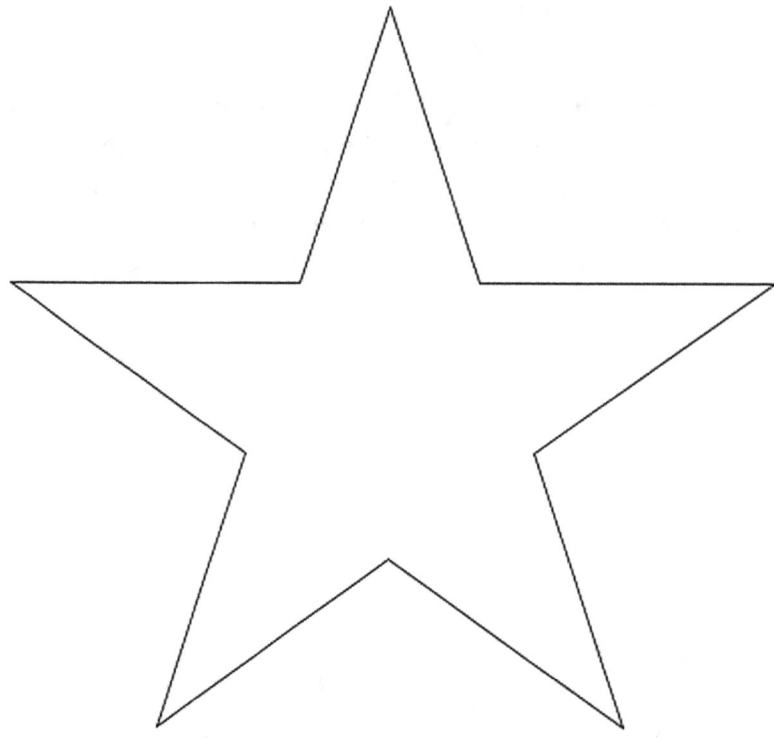

Label each of the five points of the star with a personal value that indicates what is important to you in this moment. Take a moment to center before you write, to ensure these values are an authentic representation of how you feel today. If you agree, we will share these with the group.

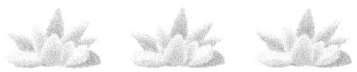

Energizing and Energy-draining Areas of Life

Awareness Activity

Name five (5) energy-draining activities, practices, or thoughts that are present in your life, and list the frequency with which they take place:

Activity   Frequency (per day/wk/mo/yr)
1.
2.
3.
4.
5.

Name five (5) energizing activities, practices, or thoughts that are present in your life, and list the frequency with which they take place:

Activity   Frequency (per day/wk/mo/yr)

1.
2.
3.
4.
5.

What have you learned about yourself and the life you've created? How can this awareness now serve you?

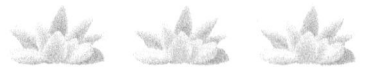

Clear Mirror, Smoky Mirror

Note:
The following activity should only be used with a well-established group that has been meeting for several months or years.

We are all wounded.

And, we are all healers.

What keeps us from knowing this about each other are the judgments we unconsciously make—about one another. Yet, healing and/or wellness is more accessible when we can transform and transcend these judgments, along with other stagnating beliefs.

How do we accomplish this?

One tool lies in the ability to see the world differently. For example, take the concept of mirrors. For the purposes of this exercise, and beyond, let us experiment with the idea that the people and experiences that present themselves are reflecting something back to us, about us.

Within each person or experience, we tend to perceive the "good" and the "not-so-good." We consciously want to identify with that which we perceive as "good," but we have resistance to the "not-so-good." Yet, if we can acknowledge that what is considered "not good" lies within us (how else would we have the ability to recognize it?), we can experience less of a sense of separation between our self and the other person.

If we can experience less separation, we find ourselves less willing to judge "the other" so harshly, which gives rise to compassion. Also, if we can identify with another person, acknowledging that whatever we perceive in them also lies within us, perhaps we can learn to have more self-compassion. This creates an opening for us to reclaim the energy we have used for judging (ourselves and others), which we can apply to creating more healing and wellness.

To do this, we must acknowledge good and "not-so-good," or what we perceive as "clear" and "smoky" within the perceived as well as the perceiver. What follows is one exercise that facilitates this experience.

Instruct members to choose a beginning partner and to sit beside them.

The team decides who will be the "giver," and who will be in the role of "receiver."

The giver begins by sitting quietly in the presence of their partner; and, recognizing that whatever they perceive in their partner is also within themselves, the "giver" verbalizes a quality that (in their perception) is "smoky" or "less desirable" or "shadow-like" in their partner. The giver says," I sometimes perceive _____ in you. This is a quality I recognize in myself, and in this way, you are my smoky mirror."

Then, the giver verbalizes a quality that (in their perception) is "clear" or "desirable" or "admirable" in their partner. The giver says," I sometimes perceive _____ in you. This is a quality I recognize in myself, and in this way, you are my clear mirror."

The receiver's job is simply to listen and receive. They may say "thank you," when the giver is finished.

Then, the giver and receiver change roles, and the exercise is begun again.

Depending on the amount of time available, and the size of the group, the exercise can be repeated until each one has partnered with everyone in the group; or, if time is limited, the exercise can be completed with a set number of members (three, five, ten, or whatever works for the group.
When everyone has completed the exercise, allow time for the group to reassemble and to share whatever they have experienced or learned from the exercise.

[At times, when I've used this exercise, group members have asked to revisit it at a later time].

A Letter to the Self

MATERIALS: Paper for letters, stamped envelopes, pens

Begin this exercise after the group meditation and check-in time.

Pass out the stamped envelopes and ask each attendee to write their home address. Pass out the paper. Instruct them to hold on to the envelopes into which they will deposit and seal their letters when done.

Now ask members to choose and sit with a partner. Once settled, bring up the subject matter of the letter they will write. Choose from the following themes:

-Something they would like to implement in their lives
-Something they would like to change
-Some unfinished business they would like to address

Ask them to close their eyes for five minutes (you may choose to play light, soft music during this time, or not) during which time you would like for them to choose one of the themes. Once they know what they want to address, they can open their eyes and convey this choice to their partner. The partner may listen and ask questions about how this change will serve their life journey. (This allows the speaker to realize his or her motivation for change). Possible questions the partner may ask include:

What will it look like for you to do this?
Who else is involved?
When will you do this?
What are the benefits of doing this?
After you've done this, how will you feel?

Allow five to ten minutes for this discussion, after which time the partners switch roles. Repeat this part of the exercise.

When the exchange is complete, ask all participants to close their eyes and use their imagination to project themselves into the future, to a time when they have accomplished their goal. Ask them to experience what their life is like in this reality, focusing on sights, sounds, scents, energy levels, happiness or relief levels, etc. (five to ten minutes). Just before counting up from one to five, ask participants to visualize a very clear final picture of 'life after the goal has been accomplished.'

Count them up from one to five and ask them to open their eyes. Once their eyes are open, ask them to write a letter from the perspective of the future self (the one who has accomplished their targeted goal) to the current self (the one undergoing the exercise). Ask participants to seal the letter in the envelope and to pass them to the facilitator, who will mail the letters one to three months later. Inform members of when to expect the letters.

The facilitator mails the letters at the appointed time, and allows time for discussion, reports and feedback at the meeting following receipt of the letters.

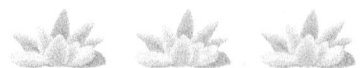

Committing to More Health and Well-Being

Instructions for the Exercise

Over the years, we've come to accept the idea that it takes twenty-one days to create a new habit or change a behavior. However, most people do not know from whence comes this idea. This thought form is actually based in science, starting with the man who wrote the book *Psycho-Cybernetics*, Dr. Maxwell Maltz.

Apparently, Dr. Maltz was originally a plastic surgeon, who noticed that it took twenty-one days for amputees to lose the sensation of a phantom limb. Dr. Maltz also observed that if his plastic surgery patients still had a negative self-image after undergoing surgery to alter the cause of this image, he could assist them with developing a new self-image within that twenty-one–day timeframe. Further observations solidified his theory about behavior change. After he wrote *Psycho-Cybernetics*, Dr. Maltz's theory found its way into our common culture and our understanding about how to create change.

Psycho-Cybernetics had no direct bearing upon the creation of this exercise, except that the theories found therein are embedded in our collective consciousness. (I created this exercise without ever knowing the origins of the twenty-one–day theory until years after this exercise had been used in numerous workshops.)

Specifics

Instruct participants to choose a partner. If an odd number of participants exists, the facilitator can partner with someone or ask for volunteers to become a group of three. Pass out the worksheets. (Make as many copies as you need.)

Instruct the partners to exchange phone numbers or e-mail addresses, to become allies for change. Similar to many programs where members are going to transcend old habits (alcoholism, eating disorders, etc.), partners will advocate for each other, provide a listening ear, etc.

Mention to participants that we all have areas of our lives that could use some improvement, and if we can find the strength and consistency to shift away from behaviors that no longer serve our "wellness journey," we can reclaim the energy from the old behaviors to enjoy new ones. Instruct participants that they are to think of three (3) commitments that they would like to make, that will contribute to their health and/or well-being. One way to do this is to have participants close their eyes while you play soft, contemplative music, and have them walk through their lives, witnessing what is unhealthy and what needs to change. For eight to ten minutes, ask them to examine:

> Relationships
> Finances
> Diet and exercise
> Mental and emotional health
> Stress levels
> The presence of, or lack of, play, relaxation, and passion
> Unfulfilled desires
> Their physical living environment

With one minute to go, ask everyone to finish surveying their lives. Ask them to open their eyes as you count up from one to three, and count them up (One…two… three…Open your eyes).

Allow a minute or two for them to integrate the information they received as they surveyed their personal lives, then have each one fill out the worksheet. If you like, you may play some music while they complete this task. Allow fifteen minutes for this.

When each one is finished, have the partners share what they've written. This is the beginning of the empowerment process. Allow eight to ten minutes, then switch, so that the listener becomes the speaker.

Close the exercise with a brief visualization: Ask participants to close their eyes and experience the sights, scents, feelings and sounds of the life with the changes already in place. Have participants see a final picture, and ask them to "turn up the intensity of light in that picture." Do not give further explanation: everyone instinctively knows what this means and how to do it. By not giving further instruction or information, you remove yourself from influencing their experience. This is important.

Count participants up from the exercise. (Say: "I'm now going to count up from one to five; and when you hear the number five, open your eyes, knowing that the picture you've just seen is the reality you are creating for yourself and will exist in some form twenty-one days from now").

Instruct partners to decide whether they will advocate for one another daily, every few days, or weekly.

Instruct participants to perform some of the actions they've listed to create the three changes written at the top of the worksheet, each and every day for twenty-one days.

If meetings are monthly, set aside time at the beginning of the next meeting for feedback and sharing about this exercise.

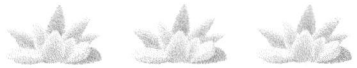

Committing to More Health and Well-Being

Name: _____   Date:

Name three (3) commitments that you can make to yourself, that will contribute to your health and/or well-being.

1. _____

2. _____

3. _____

For each commitment, list two (2) specific actions you will take to honor your commitment, and work toward actualizing the changes you want to make.

Commitment 1

    1.

    2.

Commitment 2

    1.

    2.

Commitment 3

    1.

    2.

List two (2) people, places, or groups that will support your desire to create more health and well-being.

    1.

    2.

List the characteristics of how you/your life will be, or what you will gain once these commitments have produced the desired results.

    1.   4.

    2.   5.

    3.   6.

Conversation with the Body

This exercise uses the creative imagination to open a subjective dialogue between mind and body regarding an enhancement of wellness. Participants will choose partners and will divide their time between playing the roles of speakers (the ones having the experience) and listeners (the ones guiding the experience for the speakers). Please allow fifteen to twenty minutes to complete each role, with a five- to ten-minute break before switching roles.

As an adaptation, the exercise can be managed without partners as a group experience guided by the facilitator. The facilitator would simply read the part of the listener for the entire group while each member focused on his or her own experience.

Before beginning, have participants choose a partner and locate a semiprivate space in the meeting area. Once settled into their space, have participants establish rapport with their partners. This can be accomplished by sharing a brief "check-in." Each one can take turns expressing how his or her life appears to be going in the present moment. The listener is completely dedicated to listening while the speaker shares. After a set period, the listener and speaker change places. An alternative approach would be to have each pair answer one of the questions in the "Openings" section of this book.

Once the sharing has concluded, have partners decide which is to be the speaker and which will serve as the listener.

Listeners: "Are you ready to begin?"

Once speakers answer affirmatively, listeners ask speakers to close their eyes and take in three deep, relaxing breaths, giving themselves the command to relax more deeply with each breath.

Utilizing a soft voice and a backwards count from ten to one, listeners assist speakers with moving deep inside their bodies, instructing speakers to shrink down in size, enter their body, and find themselves somewhere within…

Listeners listen with intention, only asking open questions designed to assist speakers' process—remaining silent if there is no need for assistance.

Listeners: "Now that you're inside your body, you can really communicate with it, and you can listen easily and effortlessly to what it wants to tell you.

"Tell your body, 'I've noticed a change in you lately. I've noticed that you….' " (Listen to speakers as they finish the thought.)

Listeners: "Ask the body, 'What do you want me to know?' " (Listen.)

Listeners: "Say to the body: 'How can we work together to make sure you function at the highest level?' " (Listen—if necessary, listeners can ask for more by saying, "Could you say more about that?" or "Is there more?")

Listeners: "Take a moment or two to make an agreement to work with the body. Notice everything you can about the agreement—in words, images, and feelings. Notice what you are doing to help the body function at its highest level…and notice how the body responds. Create a very clear image about this agreement…and when you've done that, raise your finger or thumb, or nod your head, as a signal that you have a clear image and/or feeling about the agreement." (Listeners allow a few minutes for Speakers to complete the task, and indicate that they are finished.)

Listeners: "Now, allow yourself to receive a gift from the body, as a symbol of the wellness you will both experience when you work together. Know that you can effortlessly receive this symbol, and that it will simply appear. Once you've received it, please raise a thumb or finger, or nod your head." (Listeners wait for the signal.)

Listeners: "Now I'm going to count up from one to five…and when you hear the number five, open your eyes and remember everything that has just happened."

Listeners and speakers sit quietly for a few moments, so that speakers can assimilate the experience. Listeners may ask how the experience was for the speaker, or may ask if there is anything the speaker would like to share about the exercise.

The facilitator notices when everyone has returned their awareness to the room and provides five minutes for speakers to share the experience with their listeners.

The facilitator creates a "state break" (a diversion from the previous state of mind), such as a stretch, a bathroom break, or an opportunity to get a drink of water. Then, switch the process: listeners and speakers change places, and the exercise begins again.

When both sides have completed the exercise, the facilitator provides an opportunity for group sharing and suggests that, if possible, it might be helpful to maintain awareness about the agreement by finding a physical representation of the gift; an object that exists in the world. If they find such an object, it will serve as a "physical anchor" or "touchstone," which may be a helpful reminder about the agreement with the body. Such an object may be helpful, but is not necessary.

Soul Cards

Some of the most magical, empowering times that transpired in the wellness group I facilitated for thirteen years occurred on nights when we disallowed preconceived ideas about the activities we "should" pursue. We sometimes experimented with ways to access unacknowledged issues and ideas about how to address them. Additionally, we engaged in activities that allowed us to recognize our strengths, wisdom, and abilities. Sometimes, we simply allowed the subconscious to speak in a safe, empowering environment. One of the tools we used to accomplish this was the "Soul Cards."

What are Soul Cards? I like the interpretation of Joan Borysenko, PhD, who said: "Each card is a stunning archetype that speaks directly to the soul. Like windows into our deepest self, these magnificent cards are an invitation to profound self-discovery."

I like to use Soul Cards (I've used Soul Cards 2) because they present evocative, archetypal images without words or interpretation, creating a clean canvas that helps individuals speak the contents of their subconscious minds. This activity is useful and healing when there is a need to lighten up, when the group energy feels stuck, or to create an opportunity for people to simply embody a different attitude. It can stand on its own, or serve as a segway to other activities during the meeting.

Materials

1 pack Soul Cards (or other archetypal cards with images)
1 basket or container, in which to pass the cards

I've utilized two methods for sparking conversations with the cards.

Method 1: (similar to the instructions in the Soul Card instructions)

Place the cards facedown in the basket or container.

After the group check-in and/or contemplative practice, have participants get in touch with a current area of challenge or concern in their lives.

Advise participants that you will pass around the Soul Cards and that they are to pick one from the pile. Ask them to accept the card they've chosen as an opportunity to receive communication from their inner self—an opportunity to give themselves permission to reflect on their lives from a different perspective.

Give participants time to view the card and reflect on the meaning it bears for them.

Ask if anyone would like to share his or her interpretations, and allow time for group sharing.

Method 2:

After a contemplative practice and/or group check-in, pass the cards around, instructing each participant to pick one, turn it over, and reflect inwardly on any meaning it bears. Do not give any more instruction. Allow a couple of minutes for people to view their card and reflect on it's meaning.

Ask people to open-mindedly, open-heartedly share their perceptions.

Significant Others
Honor Each Other

MATERIALS: Enough roses, or other flowers, for each participant—group members and significant others.

Throughout our years of meetings, we would periodically invite significant others to join our circle. The formats for these meetings were simple but powerful, according to the participants:

Begin with a group meditation (ten to fifteen minutes).

Individual introductions:

Each person in the group introduces him/herself. You may request a specific format for this, choosing some of the following parameters: name, participant or significant other of (blank); occupation; what's most inspirational about their significant other; length of relationship; etc.; or, create your own unique format. Depending on the size of the group, this may take thirty to forty-five minutes.

Honoring each other:

Inform the couples that after you provide instructions, they will find a semiprivate space to interact. Instruct them to give the rose to their significant other, as they say:

"I want to honor you because of (or for) [blank]." They have ten minutes to share memories of special or inspirational times, and to express their gratitude. Speakers express whatever they want within the theme. Receivers don't say anything or correct any perception; nor do they discount what is being said in any way. They simply listen and receive. When Speakers are finished, Receivers may thank them.

The Facilitator remains aware of the time and at the end of ten minutes asks participants to switch positions. The previous Speaker now becomes the Receiver, and the process repeats—starting with new Speakers presenting their significant others with a rose, and saying: "I want to honor you because of (or for) [blank]."

After ten minutes, the Facilitator calls everyone back to the circle. Once reassembled, the Facilitator asks if anyone has anything to share. Allow time for sharing, and end the session with the Healing Light Visualization. Thank the significant others for coming before adjourning.

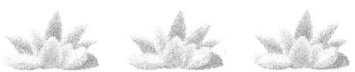

Notes

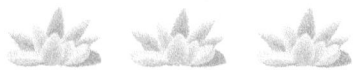

Resources

Contemplative Practices

Mindfulness Meditation

University of Massachusetts Worcester Campus
Center for Mindfulness
Mailing address: 55 Lake Avenue North
Worcester, Massachusetts 01655
Phone: 508-856-2656
http://www.umassmed.edu/cfm/home/index.aspx

Thich Nhat Hanh
Plum Village
Le Pey 24240
Thenac FRANCE
http://www.plumvillage.org/

Naropa University
2130 Arapahoe Avenue
Boulder, CO 80302-6697
303-444-0202
http://www.naropa.edu/

Jon Kabat-Zinn
(See: University of Massachusetts Center for Mindfulness)

Other Contemplative Practices

Transcendental Meditation
1-888-LEARN TM (1-888-532-7686)
http://www.tm.org/ (no physical address via Web site)

Primordial Sound
The Chopra Center
2013 Costa del Mar Rd.
Carlsbad, CA 92009
888-736-6895
http://www.chopra.com/

Surat Shabda Yoga (Light and Sound)
MasterPath
P.O. Box 9035
Temecula, CA 92589 - 9035 USA
http://www.masterpath.org

Christian Contemplative Practice via Father Thomas Keating
Contemplative Outreach, Ltd.
10 Park Place, 2nd Floor
Suite B
Butler, New Jersey 07405
973-838-3384
http://www.contemplativeoutreach.org/site/PageServer

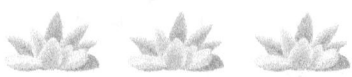

Books

Kabat-Zinn, Jon. Full Catastrophe Living: Using the Wisdom of Your Body and Mind to Face Stress, Pain, and Illness. Piatkus, London 1996. ISBN: 0-749-915-854

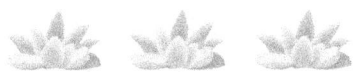

Audio

Visualization/Meditation

Belleruth Naparstek
Guided visualization CDs
http://www.healthjourneys.com/

Jon Kabat-Zinn
"Guided Mindfulness Meditation"
Available at amazon.com

Music for visualization, meditations, etc.

Peter Kater & Carlos Nakai
Migration
Natives

Bobby McFerrin
Circle Songs
Medicine Man, especially the song "Common Threads"

Steve Halpern
In the Key of Healing

Spiritual Environment
Healing
Shamanic Dream, especially the song "Shamanic Dream"

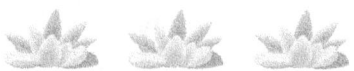

Other Resources

Soul Cards
http://www.touchdrawing.com/3SoulCards/SCmain.html

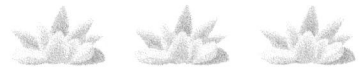

Index

www.ingramcontent.com/pod-product-compliance
Lightning Source LLC
Chambersburg PA
CBHW081416280526
45788CB00009B/3122

* 9 781453 679906 *